To me, life is about resiliency and reaching out, and remaining stalwart as one experiences the many uninvited guests that challenge that resiliency.
—*Mary Mahony*

In this amazing book, Mary Mahony describes how her resiliency was challenged by discovering at age 50 she had multiple sclerosis. Using this disease as her goad, Mary focused on her bucket list of adventures, with gratitude to her high school being at the top of the list. In characteristic fashion and with persistence, she engaged classmates and the principal to hold the first-ever all-class reunion and establish an alumni association at the school where she had developed her talents and friendships. As a lifelong educator, Mary appreciated the importance of schools in forming and refining the character of their students. In her own words:

If you went to a good high school, as I did, it truly gave you legs to follow your dreams. If you went on to college or pursued additional training, it prepared you to stand on those legs. So many times the colleges are the recipients of all the good will and the high schools are long forgotten.

Not so with Mary. Her illness provided the catalyst for finding a way to thank the many teachers and classmates who made her high school experience so rich and fulfilling. At the same time, this book encourages M.S. patients and others to focus on what they can do, rather than on what their challenges preclude. Her life and her book provide an inspiration for all of us.

As Superintendent of the Belmont Public Schools for twenty years, I have known Mary Mahony as a dedicated teacher, supportive parent, and champion of students. This book has given me a much better insight into her values and her ability to overcome challenges. It is a must-read for educators and for those who confront physical challenges every day.

Peter Holland, Ed.D.
Belmont Public Schools, Superintendent, 1988–2008

The journey of each patient with multiple sclerosis (M.S.) is different, and Mary has wonderfully captured this in *The Reunion, Warm Regards, M.S.* It describes her unique perspective on this neurologic disease and how it has affected her life, creating challenges and opportunities. M.S. needs many such voices for it to be understood in all of its complexity, and *The Reunion* is an important element of the tapestry of life experiences that emerge from a diagnosis of M.S.

Using the old analogy of life as a slowly flowing river, the initial biological events that trigger the altered immune responses in M.S. are a powerful but largely invisible current below a placid surface, and it is only a decade or more later that symptoms may emerge to the surface and lead to a diagnosis. The resulting ripples through a patient's life and that of her family are just as complex as the biology of M.S. that we are only beginning to understand.

And just as we treat M.S. to control the behavior of the immune system, patients can influence the repercussions of a diagnosis on their lives. Whether patients have a benign or severe course to their M.S., I have always been struck by their resilience and their ability to turn the tables and use this life experience to transform themselves and not be defined by their biology. I thank Mary for sharing this story with me, and hope it inspires many other patients to relate their M.S. journeys.

Philip L. De Jager, M.D., Ph.D.
Steven R. & Kathleen P. Haley Distinguished Chair for the Neurosciences
Director of the Program in Translational NeuroPsychiatric Genetics
Departments of Neurology and Psychiatry
Brigham & Women's Hospital
Associate Professor of Neurology, Harvard Medical School
Associate Member, Broad Institute of Harvard and MIT

The Reunion,

WARM REGARDS, M.S.

The Reunion,

WARM REGARDS, M.S.

Mary Mahony

REDDING PRESS·BELMONT, MA

Susan A. Pasternack, Editor
Portrait on back of book by Carol Evans Photography, Boston, MA

Non-Fiction

ISBN 13: 9780965887977
ISBN: 0965887979
Library of Congress Control Number: 2016957211
Redding Press

Dedication

To the one classmate who believed that, together, we could realize a dream.

To the amazing school principal and committee members who supported us so that the dream could come true.

To the Class of '66 and those who came before and after.

To all who believe that there is good karma in a bucket list.

To my amazing mother, who never knew I had M.S.

To all who have M.S.

May they someday find a cure.

Life is like an adventure park. Each person gets only one ticket to enter. Sometimes we are up for the ride, while other times we might prefer to pass. Once it starts, there is no getting off. It can be a wonderful ride, or scary as hell. Most important, we try to get it all in before closing time.

Mary Mahony

The Attack

For years I had been keeping a mental note of all the things that I hadn't gotten to but wanted to do in my lifetime. I guess we now call such account settling our "bucket lists." My bucket list had long included a number of people, places, and organizations I wanted to repay in one way or another. So, after years of working hard as an educator, writer, wife, and mother, I was ready to start paying back. It was time for me to turn my bucket list from an intellectual exercise into my very own life series.

Never did I imagine that at the age of fifty all those reckonings would become the start of a new chapter of my life. The scene began very early one May morning. My life changed dramatically that day. I remember lying in my bed and feeling nothing on the right side of my body. It was as if someone had sliced me right down the middle: the left side was fine, but the right side, from the top of my head to the tips of my toes, had suddenly been taken away from me. The feeling seemed surreal and was the closest I had ever come to an out-of-body experience. I felt absolutely powerless as a tear came trickling down my left cheek. It was the first time in my life that I was crying on only one side of my face. And as I lay there wiping away my tear, I had the daunting thought that I was only one week away from getting on a plane and attending my husband's thirtieth college reunion at the

White House, since President Bill Clinton was in his class. It was to be an amazing celebration. I wondered how I would get out of the bed, let alone travel on a plane to Washington, D.C.

I cannot begin to recount the emotions I felt in those first few moments. It was as if I was being held hostage by my own body. I knew immediately that the life I had known was gone. I remember going from a sense of fear of the unknown, to one of loss and sadness, and, finally, to determination and gratitude that this episode was being experienced by me and not by one of my children.

It was hard to imagine that at a mere fifty years of age, in the blink of an eye, my whole life had changed, and I had absolutely nothing to do with it. Getting out of bed was my first hurdle. I rolled out and literally fell flat on my face. My left side was on the inside of the bed and of no help to me whatsoever. My right side was the one that had been affected, the side that I depended on each morning to exit my bed and begin my day. And because that part of me was not functioning, the expression "she doesn't have a leg to stand on" suddenly took on a whole new meaning.

When I finally got myself into the bathroom, nothing happened. One side of my body was in another time zone. That was the scariest moment, as I sat there wondering if my bodily functions would ever return to normal. Things continued to go downhill when somehow I managed to enter the shower. As the water streamed down, I felt as if needles were pelting the nerves in my back. The pain was excruciating.

Long before I ever saw a doctor, I knew what I had: multiple sclerosis. I remember sitting down at my desk the day after my attack and going online to explore how it might continue to manifest itself once I recovered from this episode. The medical education I got in those early days was one that I would have preferred to skip. Very late one night soon after the attack, I massaged and prioritized my bucket list, as well as penned the first entry in a journal that I continue to keep today. As important as all the things that I still wanted to experience were the paybacks to all the people and places that so richly deserved some of my time and energy. Having served on any number of boards and organizations that surely deserved an infusion of my energy, the top line item that would eventually become the beneficiary of my skills would be my former high school. In hindsight, I think I have those people and places on my bucket list to thank, and then some, because they became my finish line. The race was on!

Fast-forward thirteen years: I had full bodily function, was totally vertical, and presented with few visible reminders of that awful May morning. Here I was standing on top of the hill outside my old high school scanning a field that had been divided into fifty blocks, one for each graduating class. This gathering was a dream realized.

Before me were some 600 people representing a span of the school's fifty classes of graduates. It was as if time had stood still and I was once again a high school student, although my peers were greying at the temples and in some cases not moving quite so quickly or easily as I remembered. As I watched the emotion-filled embraces, I could hear the laughter echo all the way up to the top of the hill. Standing next to me was my classmate and co-conspirator in this day's festivities. Like me, she had fully believed that we could pull this off. What I had dreamed of for so many years had finally come true. And what was once a line item was happening right before my eyes.

My reason for originally creating the bucket list didn't matter anymore. The image of the one scene that I kept replaying, the one that had drawn me back all those years, would soon be a rerun; finally, it was all there in front of me. For that one day I felt as if my classmates and I had gone from being teenagers to senior citizens all in an instant. As I continued to watch the celebration, my mind drifted back to all those years before, the long-ago past that had inspired this special day.

The Move

THERE MAY HAVE BEEN ANY number of reasons why my parents chose to move to the country and leave the pleasures of a large town, none of which I was privy to at the time. They left behind the convenience of living right above a beautiful Atlantic beach, with very easy train access to New York City, to relocate to a small country town almost forty-five minutes away. We were going from a half acre of land to two acres, from having four grocery store chains to choose from to only two country stores, and from the delights of a movie theatre, playhouse, and bustling town center that met our every need to some less impressive and somewhat limited retail offerings.

I was given hardly any notice about the move; it felt more like packing and being dropped off a fast-moving truck. Our old house sold almost immediately, and no sooner had my school year ended than it was bye-bye beach and hello brooks. No longer would I pass the house where my great-grandmother had once lived or the one that belonged to my grandparents, which I saw on my way to the bus stop each morning. No longer would I enjoy the bed of white violets or the scent of my great-grandmother's almond bush in spring. No longer would I smell baking bread and homemade pies as I played underneath the old cherry tree that I so loved. No longer would I spend my sick days on my grandmother's couch being pampered with her homemade chicken soup or the meals we shared at my grandparents' table. Never again could I say that I went to the same schools that my dad had attended. And never again could I walk half a mile to bask in the sun on a beach on Long Island Sound, one frequented by the rich and famous as they pulled their yachts into their slips. I can still remember seeing Elizabeth Taylor and Eddie Fisher as well as Paul Newman, Darren McGavin, Tony Randall, Imogene Coca, and Sid Caesar, all names that mean nothing to the stargazers of today.

For a fourth grader, moving was not as easy as it would have been for a kindergartner and perhaps not as hard as it would be for a seventh grader. I had been redistricted after third grade, so in reality the classmates I was leaving behind I had only known for a year. Even so, I was very sad to be saying goodbye to much of my extended family as well as to the only place I had ever called home.

Adjusting

OUR NEW LIFE IN A secluded corner in the country reminded me more of life in the little towns in rural New England, where you were not a few streets away from your friends but acres apart. I felt as if I were in a foreign country, even though I was really not far from where I used to live. Although my parents hoped that their enthusiasm for this new area was contagious, that was not the case at all.

Our country house was brand-new and situated in a cul-de-sac that had eight other houses scattered about like dots on a map; there seemed to be a lot more land than houses. Our house faced a wonderful farm, and I remember looking through binoculars and seeing the cows wandering along the hills below. That farm, much like something out of a Norman Rockwell painting, was about ten acres away from our new house.

There are small towns and then there are very small towns, and I soon found out that in our neighborhood the centers of activity were poles apart and yet the distance in between was, in reality, very little. As you entered the local market, people were almost overly accommodating, and you instantly felt as if you were with old friends. Instead of fifteen aisles as before, there were now only four, and you could see all the way to the back of the store when you entered the front door. One of my earliest memories is of viewing the whole side of a cow hanging from a hook as the butcher asked my mom what cut she wanted. That was a new sight for me! Across the street from the grocery store was a pizza parlor, owned by a man not known for employing the best hygiene. That was a very short-lived experience for us. Rather sad for me, since I loved pizza.

Next to the grocery store was the local bar, and word had it that if your husband did not come home from work on time, the local bar was the first place you might look to find him. In truth, it was the local watering hole, where problems were shared and I am sure many creative suggestions were offered.

A short distance down the road was the lumberyard, and adjacent to that a dry goods store, where you could pick up everything from underwear to toothpicks, a remnant of a whole other era. Then across the street from that was the post office. These were all family businesses, so everyone was related by either marriage or genetics. In every way we were outsiders, but never did we feel treated as such.

By far the most impressive piece of property in the area was a large wire mill that employed about 75 percent of the people who lived nearby. I would venture to say that anyone in the Northeast and beyond who bought wire from the early 1900s to about 1985 would have found that it was made in that mill. It was a massive place, and had been there for years and years, a magnet for many of the businesses that had been set up around it.

If you liked penny candy and wanted a lesson in local history, you stopped into Ma K's store. The store was so dark that when you entered you thought the place was closed, until Ma Kearns appeared. The only thing older than the candy was Ma K herself, a tiny woman with wire-rimmed glasses who was barely five feet tall and welcomed you with her sweet smile and raspy voice each time you entered her store. When she stood behind the candy counter you could hardly see her mouth. Somewhere in the background was her husband, and later her son, but none of them seemed to matter. It was all about Ma Kearns, who had a heart bigger than the whole town. Ma K knew everything about everyone, and of course we were immediately interrogated the first time we stopped there. The candy shop was always the last place we visited after we picked up our groceries. Eventually, a drugstore opened a stone's throw from Ma K's candy store, but that came some time later.

Last, but not least, was the gas station, both the first thing you saw when you entered town or the last thing you passed when you left. The lady who pumped your gas was also a second-grade teacher in our local elementary school. Her husband owned the gas station and worked long hours, so I guess that's how they bonded. The wife was tall and lanky and had long ringlets, like Little Lulu. It always impressed me that she could pull off being an adult while sporting a child's hairdo. The couple were as delightful and welcoming as everyone else and made getting your gas pumped a very social experience.

We lived on the west side of the town, where there was another small grocery store, a post office, a liquor store, eventually a drugstore, and a country emporium, as well as a train station. If you crossed over the train tracks and down the road a bit, you arrived at a pond that, once frozen, was the focal point of many wonderful winter nights of ice skating, always with a crackling fire burning to warm your hands and feet. Although the town was the polar opposite from the one I had just left, it had a certain charm that intrigued me, even when I was a ten-year-old child. But I was not about to tell my parents that I almost liked our new hometown.

By our third visit to the grocery store, everyone who worked there knew our names, where we lived, where we had moved from, whose land we built our house on, and how long we intended to stay. It was not as if someone was pumping you for information but more a spirit of "neighborliness," which made you feel right at home and no longer a newcomer. It was clear that everyone truly wanted you to like living there, and even more important, were glad you had come.

In this town, life was certainly all about wheels, and everything you did not drive to pick up was delivered. Our bakery goods were brought by a bread man three times a week. Our milk came daily, and our knives were sharpened by a craftsman whose truck resembled a small hardware store on wheels. Doors were never locked and neighbors dropped in at all hours, sometimes bringing a wonderful edible treat. Other times they would arrive and enjoy a late drink. In summer, there were many neighborhood picnics, each at a different person's house. Everything you ate was farm fresh and homemade and absolutely delicious.

Our home was one of the typical ranch houses that could be found all over New England at the time. My parents had had it built for our family, and it was surrounded by a blanket of green grass that went on for as far as the eye could see. My mom often chastised my dad for making the yard so massive. He had to purchase a riding mower to do the job, and that got old so quickly that he even tried to convince me to ride it and mow the lawn. "In your dreams," I thought to myself.

I spent most of the first few weeks in my new neighborhood riding the used bicycle that my dad had bought me from the Western Auto store. I had never been allowed to ride a bike where we used to live, since the road was very busy and we were on a blind curve. It was a big deal when my dad conceded and reluctantly agreed to allow me to have a bike, but of course not a new one. It was truly my only form of entertainment that first summer. In hindsight, I think that's probably why my dad agreed to let me have it. I would ride it around the circle in our cul-de-sac until I was almost dizzy. Then I would head on down to the brook to talk to the frogs, with whom I shared some very heavy stuff over the years. I surely would have "croaked" if they had reported any of it.

Country Living 101: Don't rub elbows with the poison ivy. Did I ever look like someone from outer space, with eyes so swollen that I had mere slits for seeing and legs that were covered with bubbling blisters that oozed and itched all at the same time. If that wasn't bad enough, while I was healing I decided to pick blueberries one day and stepped on a yellow jacket's nest. Off to the hospital I went, sans blueberries.

Perhaps the hardest part of moving at this time of the year was that my cousin, who vacationed at the beach and whom I saw daily in summer, as well as my friends, were back where we used to live. I envied them for still being by the ocean and enjoying all the things that we did each summer. I felt very lonely and out of place in our new surroundings. I often wandered next door to visit a couple who were about ten years younger than my own parents and had a very active house. Childless in those early days, they embraced me; I truly felt as if I had a second family. They became my anchor when I was floating around the neighborhood, and have continued to be my role models for most of my life. When I wasn't riding my bike or talking to the frogs, I would find myself on their doorstep.

Instead of hearing the relentless beach traffic or the golfers hitting their balls at the driving range as before, my nights were very still in the country and the silence was deafening. I welcomed the summer katydids and the sound of the bullfrogs as they croaked their way through the night. But on a hot night, I missed the ocean breeze that would find its way to our old house. In its place was an oppressive, humid heat that could only be relieved with the assistance of a very noisy fan.

I enjoyed those first weekends after we moved when we would go back to see my grandmother and spend a bit of time at the beach, but it wasn't *my* beach anymore. The wonderful games of hide-and-seek in the evenings, after a day spent in the ocean, were a mere memory. In just a few short weeks everything had changed, and I felt a sense of loss that I had never known before. There were no girls on our new street or for that matter anywhere near our new house. The only kid in my new neighborhood was a boy, and I had no interest in hanging out with him. Books became my friends for the summer, and I would lie and read in our hammock for hours and hours.

Back to School

YOU CAN ONLY IMAGINE THAT the start of school that first fall did not come soon enough for me. Although I was a bit anxious, I looked forward to meeting my new teacher and making new friends. We had visited the school when my mom registered me and were met at the door by the principal, Mr. G., who was so tall that he reminded me of the man on stilts at the circus. He was also stern-looking and his bushy eyebrows created a visor for his deep-set eyes. But he was very welcoming while simultaneously warning me that he carried a ruler with him at all times.

I was impressed by how small the school was compared to the one I had left, which had five tracks per grade. My new school had two, and sometimes three tracks, and I would be in a class of only fifteen students rather than twenty-two. I certainly hoped I liked them, because if I didn't, there would be very slim pickings.

I remember that first day of school, my fifth-grade year, as if it were happening right now. My teacher fit the stereotype of the old school marm to a T. She was very matronly looking, very grey, with skin like corduroy. I felt as if my grandmother had become my teacher. She immediately commented on the fact that my last name was very long and that in the interest of time, it might be better to simply put Mary S. on my papers. So for that year we would both be Miss S., and I totally appreciated her allowing me to do this. Miss S. was as warm and wonderful as she was strict, and she worked hard to connect me with the girls in my class to make me feel welcome. I recall becoming almost instant friends with the girl who sat next to me in class, and I had a playdate with her within days of starting school.

School kept me quite busy, and I loved that I could do additional writing projects and earn extra credit. Miss S. knew right from the beginning that I loved to write, and she often complimented me not only on the content of my writing but also on my penmanship. I actually think it was my time with her that made me realize that writing opened up a whole new world, a world that could be concretely real or abstractly unreal. I regret that I never saved any of the stories that I wrote that first year.

I wish that I could say that I had the same positive experience with the school's music teacher. Although I was never able to hold a note, I always enjoyed singing at home. Even when I sat by the brook, I would serenade the frogs. In my mind, I knew I was no Karen Carpenter, but I never dreamed I would be asked *not* to sing at all. That is exactly what happened when Mrs. H., the music teacher, who may have known a lot about music but nothing about self-esteem and feelings, asked me to sing "Oh Aunt Lucy, why don't you ring that bell." High notes were not my strength. My bell went to hell in a hand basket, as Mrs. H. looked at me very sternly and announced in front of my entire class that I would be the person drawing the curtain for the school play and not singing a note. I could feel the tears welling up in my eyes and was immediately rescued by Miss S., who asked me to run an errand to the office for her. As much as I loved music, and still do, I have to say this single act made me feel musically impaired for the rest of my life. Years later, when I became an educator, that experience made me advocate strongly for all my students when it came to music. I am happy to report that all my own children are musically inclined and some have continued to play an instrument into their adult life. My six-year-old granddaughter is now taking voice lessons while her sister is studying the recorder. And, of course, a line item on my bucket list was music, and so at the age of sixty I began taking piano lessons and continue to do so as I write.

I made amazing friends at that little school and I actually had more fun than I had ever had where I lived before. The students came from interesting backgrounds and I loved meeting all their families. Some were blue-collar workers like my own dad, while others were professionals. But that was all unimportant. I remember one friend who lived in a house that had a spiral staircase leading to her parents' bedroom. We often played on the staircase and would pretend we were movie stars making our debut. My friend moved away about a year after I met her. A lifetime later, she also became a writer, although her subject matter is a bit more explicit and for adults only and not at all akin to mine.

I had my first male teacher when I was a sixth grader. Mr. M. was bald, wore period tortoise-shell glasses over very small eyes, and looked like a professor. Not unlike Miss S., he, too, was a fabulous teacher and totally devoted to math and science. I learned to love science in a way that I never had before. I vividly remember the plant project I created for the school science fair and the award I received for my work. It is clear to me now that the fair made a dramatic difference in how I viewed science from then on.

In addition to being a time for learning, sixth grade was when all the girls seemed to notice the boys for the first time. There was always a buzz about who had a crush on whom. When we had little activities in the gym and needed a boy as a partner, such as for square dancing, everyone got very silly and there was a lot of blushing. I already had my eye on an "older boy" I had met ice skating the first year I moved there, but that is a story for my high school years.

At the end of sixth grade, we were all sent over to a newly formed regional high school for students from grades seven through twelve. Our town and the one next to us became the bookends to this first-ever high school for each of our towns. No longer would students have to be bused to city high schools. Now we could be educated where we lived. This collaboration was a first for the area.

I remember the afternoon that all the sixth-grade girls and boys from the other town reluctantly piled out of a bus to meet all the sixth graders from our town. Everyone just stood there checking each other out, not saying a word. Finally, the girls from my town went over and introduced themselves to the new girls, and after that the boys also started to mingle and talk. It must have been hysterical for the adult spectators to witness. Amazingly, many of the kids I met that day would later become some of my dearest friends.

Soon, elementary school was over, and I experienced a small pang of loss as I said goodbye to my wonderful teachers and the intimacy that you feel in such a small school. Even though I had only been there for two years, I truly felt a special bond with my teachers. A few of my friends were moving on to private schools or relocating, just as I had done two years before. I wished I had had a crystal ball so that I could have seen where my classmates had ended up after high school. I never dreamed way back then that someday I would find out. Even more important, I wish that I had known that many decades later, I would be checking off line items on a bucket list that included these very friends and classmates.

A Better Summer? Not!

EVERYONE HAS AT LEAST ONE summer in their young lives that was a complete bust and the summer after sixth grade was truly mine. Although I had made some great friends, I was still the new girl in town, and many of the others were involved in activities they had done together for many summers. My new friends lived far away and having a playdate became a major undertaking. In addition to the challenges of getting to my new friends, one of my biggest adjustments was no longer living near my grandparents. Shortly after we moved, my grandfather passed away, and my grandmother dearly missed not only my grandfather but having us nearby since my dad was an only child. After many lonely months, my grandmother decided to rent out her house near the beach and come and stay with us for the summer. Having her back helped to fill the void I felt when we moved away from them, but it did not satisfy my need to be with old friends. Unfortunately, it was also the hottest summer I had ever experienced, and we all missed going to my grandmother's house on the weekends and swimming in Long Island Sound. Between the heat and the boredom, I was more than ready to begin school again in the fall.

For junior high school, which was located at the high school, my bus ride was twice as long as it had been in elementary school, but I had made a friend on the bus the very first year I moved to the country and I would be met by her smiling face each time I climbed aboard. The bus ride itself was a lot of fun, in part because it had students from seventh grade all the way up to the twelfth, and it was very special being in all that good company. I have such wonderful memories of how the older students looked after us underlings. They were the ones who used to get the whole bus, including the bus driver, singing "Ninety-nine Bottles of Beer on the Wall." Surely it is the last thing kids sing on a school bus today.

The Halls of Academe

FROM THE DAY IT OPENED its doors, our new regional high school, which at the time was also my junior high, had an excellent academic rating. I cannot remember having anything but extremely competent teachers who truly loved teaching almost as much as they loved learning. It was an exciting time for our school, and an academic and social smorgasbord for any student, with great subject offerings, sports, clubs, theatre, and of course, the ever-present opportunity to make new friends. I was never at a loss for things to do, and my weekends were jam-packed. A few of our classmates had barns where they would throw parties. For me, those finished barn rooms seemed as big as a dance hall, but when I revisited them some years later, they were no larger than a studio apartment.

One Saturday a month, the area Boys' Club would have a mixer for our grade level, and kids from both towns would come together and dance to songs like "Blue Moon," "One Hundred Pounds of Clay," "My Boyfriend's Back," "Duke of Earl," and to really get you shakin', "The Twist." I especially remember watching *American Bandstand* with my friends in an attempt to improve our dancing skills and prepare for the mixers. Dick Clark made everyone want to put their dancing shoes on, and I am sure we were not the only ones watching him and learning how to shake it up.

For all the wonderful memories I enjoy from those years, there were some recollections of school that were not so good. It was a frightening time for our country. I remember the air raid drills, when we would have to get under our desks and/or put our heads down with our arms wrapped around them. Each drill was a surprise, and the teacher would guide us through it. When it was over, the teacher would explain to us once again why this was necessary. I learned about communism, what the word propaganda meant, what a cold war was, and also what a spy did. Those were heavy-duty terms, and at the time we were far too young to completely understand their global significance; our world was really the distance between our home and our school.

Summers seemed to get better and better as I got older, and there was actually quite a bit to do in the country. I loved the smell of the morning air and the sound of the birds. These were different from the smells where I had lived before, since much of that was all about the ocean and the tides. For the senses, the country had much to offer, and with each year I lived there, I grew to appreciate it more and more.

We would often play tennis or swim. Very few of my friends attended camp, and most of us hung out at friends' swimming pools. When you don't live near the beach and you are lucky enough to have the space and income, you build a swimming pool. Pool parties were the rage.

It is unfortunate that sometimes when we are young we make decisions that we regret and one of mine involved sitting on the back of my friend's brother's Harley, and herding his sheep into their barn. The family lived on a lot of acreage, so those sheep were running in all directions, with the Harley a fair distance behind. But the sound of it surely seemed nearby to the animals. At the time, I was told it was a less time-consuming way of herding the sheep into the barn and that my friend only did it when his parents were away in the city. I loved animals and thought it might be fun to join in. Most unlucky for me, my mom was not working in the city that day. She happened to be riding by the house at just the right time. I was grounded for a month, at the ripe old age of fourteen. Thankfully, Mom did not witness the sheep part! Little did my mom know that another boy, who was my age and lived in the other direction, had taught me how to drive his dad's jeep when I was twelve. Relax: We never ventured out on the road, only his fields. His family had a lot of land, his dad and mom traveled regularly, and evidently the housekeeper was not doing her job. I remember how hard we would laugh when we hit a bump. It was a pathetic-looking vehicle and all in young fun. In truth, if my own kids had done something like that I would have had a heart attack just thinking about it. Sadly, my friend in crime, who became a very successful engineer, is no longer here to enjoy this flashback with me.

My junior high years went by in a flash. By eighth grade, I was actively invested in all our school events and really looked forward to each day. Students from the two towns had bonded and it was hard to ever imagine not being in school with them. Summers were rich and full of activities complemented by a great circle of friends that spanned both towns.

Then suddenly, it seemed, I found myself a high school student. We had our own identity as freshmen, normally the bottom of the ladder. We were not treated with disdain, perhaps because we had already been there for two years. My classes were interesting; Latin and French were my favorites. I aspired to become a French teacher, so there was quite a draw not only to the subject matter but also to the entertaining teacher who taught it: Mrs. H., Madame Professeur, the most eccentric teacher I ever had and also one of the most brilliant teachers I have ever known.

Madame had the good looks of Shirley MacLaine, coupled with Bette Midler's personality and candid wit. She stood about five feet tall, with a pixie haircut and gorgeous blue eyes. She was very well dressed. I think she must have been a knockout in her college days at Smith. She always had a cigarette in her hand during class, and because this practice was absolutely prohibited, Mrs. H. would smoke out the window and point out to all of us that she was not smoking in class but rather outside of it. She would also remind us of what a tattle-tale was. A Seven Sisters graduate who had lived abroad and eventually married, she was the trip of all trips. And, boy, did we learn our French. I studied French with her all four years of high school, and years later, she even attended my wedding. She clearly had a major impact on the person I became.

It was Madame who introduced me to French plays, and each year we would perform one for the entire school and our families. I loved being on the stage and Madame made it more like an adventure than schoolwork. The sets were fantastic, as were the scripts, and there were wonderful cast parties at the end of the last performance. I remember the time I volunteered to make 200 cream puffs for one of those events. I had never made a cream puff in my life, but I learned quickly, as did my mom, and I was very lucky that she was still talking to me when we were done.

A close second to Madame was Mr. M., my Latin instructor, a brilliant teacher and a true Latin scholar. He would even dress up in a toga on Saturnalia Day. Unlike Madame, Mr. M. was very serious about his work in a different way, and I learned early on that his commitment to the success of his students went above and beyond what was expected. I was an excellent Latin student until one day, when my grade plummeted from an A to a D on one of the Latin quizzes. Mr. M. took me aside and asked what I had been doing the night before. I explained that I had been babysitting, and when he asked me why, I reported that I liked earning money. A week later he had me tutoring my peers who were failing Latin, to the tune of $5 an hour. That was an extraordinary solution; it got me to study more and provided some cheap help for my peers. And I earned a lot more tutoring Latin than I ever did babysitting. Mr. M. was an amazing educator, and in the course of a career that spanned many years, his efforts were rewarded through study supported by two Fulbright grants. I was fortunate to renew our ties right before he passed away.

My gym teacher was deeply interested in fitness, and extremely fit herself. I have wonderful memories of her cheering us on as we climbed the ropes to the ceiling of the gym or giving us the courage we needed to do a double flip on the trampoline. Never in all those years did I have any clue that she and my math teacher, also a woman, were an item. It warmed my heart to see them together years later, well into their 80s, still very much in love, and enjoying their retirement together.

I have a very vivid memory of an artist visiting and doing a presentation on El Greco when I was a high school freshman and I can even remember the exact location of the room where it took place. Years later, when I was in college studying art history, I remember how impressed my professor was that I knew so much about El Greco. I recall her asking me if perhaps we had an El Greco at home. Imagine! I think my response was that my Uncle Vic did all our artwork. He painted while he was in Florida for the winter, so most of it was palm trees with a few coconuts dangling from them, with the ocean in the background. I suppose if he had added a big hand grabbing the coconuts, it might have hinted at an El Greco.

My freshman biology teacher was all about plants and bodies. My love for anatomy developed when we dissected a variety of creatures. She had placed a fabulous skeleton by the door, which greeted us as we entered her room. I really got into dissecting, and I was quite interested in the placement of all the organs and learning how everything worked. Apparently, one of my male classmates did not share my enthusiasm, since he went from vertical to horizontal in a nanosecond and begged to be dismissed from any more of that. Although it was not at all funny when it happened, the scene was like a bit from *Saturday Night Live*, though in those days I suppose it would have been more like *Candid Camera*. First he was standing, then he started to moan, and the last thing we heard from him was "Oh geez," and he was down. That's one very creative way to get out of dissecting.

Of course the real drama that unfolded almost hour by hour was all about how the opposite sex can attract and distract all at the same time. There was always that hot buzz going around about who was hanging out with whom and whether they were actually an item or not. I found it totally entertaining, as long as it did not involve me.

There were many great guys in our class as well as in the class above us. They were not necessarily the ones that you wanted to date, but those who were interesting to talk to and fun to be with. Drugs were not on the scene, at least not yet, and so everyone came to school pretty much intact. Alcohol was certainly out there, even at our school, but many of us were having too much fun without it. And there were some interesting things going on with the faculty. For instance, our awesome art teacher was let go because he was the advisor to the school newspaper and allowed a student to write something that suggested a belief in a form of government that our country did not support. It was a hot potato at the time, and all the upperclassmen were buzzing about it. Suddenly, he was gone, not unlike some of the quick fires that happen today. But today there are powerful unions, so it is not quite as fluid as it was then.

One of my favorite English teachers was released during my sophomore year. We were reading *Hamlet* and he asked the class what a nunnery was. At the time there was a "know-it-all goody two-shoes" in our class who always had her hand waving, even before the entire question came out of the teacher's mouth. She made it a habit of shutting out anyone else who might have wanted to participate. So, of course, our teacher called on her.

"Well," she said, "a nunnery is a place where nuns live." "No, no, it is a goddamned whorehouse," he very dramatically responded, since in Elizabethan times a nunnery was indeed a brothel. Having been a college professor prior to arriving at our high school, sometimes he lost sight of what was acceptable vocabulary and that was surely one of those times. He was also the first English teacher to have a class in our high school read *Who's Afraid of Virginia Woolf.* I thought it was a remarkable piece of literature, and I also thought his teaching style matched the play. You truly felt as if you *really* were that character as you read your part. He was an inspiring educator.

Evidently the school committee did not agree, and that was the end of him. But he went out in style. On the last day of class, he packed his Volkswagen convertible with protesting students and drove it around the high school, beeping his horn and waving goodbye to the principal.

Then there were the sets of young teachers who became an item, although the students were not supposed to know. The couple would gush over each other as they passed in the hallway. In June, they would leave with two last names and return in September with only one. We played along with it all, and would always look really surprised when school began again and give them an "Oh, wow, we had no idea!"

But by far my most compelling memory of sophomore year was the assassination of President John F. Kennedy. I was in math class when our principal came on the loud speaker announcing that the president of the United States had been shot. It gives me shivers just thinking about it now. I remember my math teacher lowering his head, as tears rolled down his cheeks. I had never experienced such silence in our school building. We were immediately dismissed from class, and I joined some of my classmates who went to a local Catholic church to pray. President Kennedy had already died, but it was not until later that day that this was disclosed.

The death of President Kennedy brought our whole country together and it also brought us together as a student body in a way that nothing had before. Kids you didn't know would greet you in the hall. Who would have imagined that in the next few years, Martin Luther King and Robert F. Kennedy would suffer the same fate. These were heinous, evil crimes of hatred done by people in our own country. Never would I have imagined that years later we would see the horrific acts of 9/11 or the infamous Marathon Bombing in Boston, when an innocent child was killed as he ran back to the sidelines holding up a sign as his dad crossed the finish line. Or the Orlando nightclub shootings and explosions, when a group of people were killed because they loved each other. All are reminders to us that we are fortunate to be Americans and live in a democracy where hatred and prejudice are denounced and freedom celebrated.

The Crush

So often when people reminisce about their high school years, they remember their first crush. As I reflect on that time in my own life, I have one memory in particular that always puts a smile on my face. I had met him the first year I moved out to the country. He was so different from the others, so thoughtful, not on an ego trip, fun to be with. His family was wonderful, and I remember spending many meals at their table, a table full of laughter and fun and wonderful conversation. I can still recall the actual day of our first date and the wonderful honey balls his mom had made for Easter. We hung out at his house devouring the treats while chatting with his very funny mom. Then we took a walk outside and I remember how excited I was when he held my hand.

Long before we became an item we were friends and that was the best part. I remember doing crazy things with him, like making dinners that were take-offs of movies such as *Tom Jones*; going into New York City for the day and seeing a play; watching him in school performances; and having wonderful dinner and movie dates discussing any number of interesting topics. Once we spent a whole weekend clearing the island in the middle of his parents' pond. We looked as if we were auditioning for *Gilligan's Island.*

One of the times I remember most clearly was when he bought a used M.G. and spent a whole Saturday getting it ready so he could take me to the school dance. He forgot to check out the broken lock on the passenger door, and as a result, I had to hold the door shut with a rope while I was all decked out. None of our parents had any idea that the door was being held closed this way. When I got to the dance, I was the only person with a nice dress on and a head that looked like I had stuck my hand in a socket. Fortunately, my beautiful dress offset the blown hair. I think we laughed about it for weeks.

My favorite pastime was when we would go to a pond, located close to my house, and get in a dinghy and row around for hours, just talking. We discussed everything from school to family to our futures. It felt so comfortable to me then, but it wasn't until years later that I realized how special he had made my last years of high school. It was all in great fun, and in the end, such a healthy relationship. I feel very lucky to have spent so many years with such an amazing person and it comes as no surprise to me that he is a very successful adult and a wonderful husband to the sister of one of my high school classmates. Best of all, we are all still good friends and can now look back and laugh at those times.

I was very active in clubs in high school, in particular, the American Field Service Club and the French Club. I loved languages and assumed I would one day become a French teacher. The AFS Club was all about becoming an exchange student and going abroad for an entire school year. This was my dream, something only Madame, the club's advisor, was aware of. I remember Madame taking me aside and encouraging me to apply to the program. Although I was very excited about the adventure, I knew my dad would never agree to it. I still have this clip on my screen of life of the night I brought the subject up at dinner, when my dad gave a very quick and adamant "No!" I cannot begin to express how disappointed I was. My dad was never a person open to negotiation.

In high school I started writing more and more, and at one point was scribe for the sports section of our school newspaper. I loved writing, and I penned some of my best short stories then. We had quite an amazing English department at our school, and I attribute many of my writing skills to my teachers there. I remember being complimented my first week of college for a paper I wrote about "Summer Endings." Years later, I ran into one of my high school English teachers while I was walking across my graduate school campus. He was there working on his doctorate. I remember telling him how much I appreciated the grammar diagrams we did and the picky, picky marks teachers put on my papers, all of which pushed and encouraged me to become a better writer.

For every bump we experienced there was always something to celebrate, and for a small school we had plenty of school spirit. In only a short amount of time we had soared to the top of the academic charts. Students from surrounding towns even paid tuition to attend our school. As I write, it continues to be a very impressive school, and in many ways, even better than when we were students there.

But these were times for experimentation, especially by teenagers, and we did have one drug popular at our school and that was alcohol. We lived in a small town with narrow, winding roads. There were no street lights to illuminate the way if you were speeding or under the influence. Even when you were sober, sometimes an overactive deer would decide to challenge your driving skills.

One of the girls I befriended was a cheerleader who possessed a whole school full of spirit in one tiny body. She was an only child, and her parents were both employed by our school system. They had been married several years before having her, and in every way she was the light of their lives. That light went dark on her boyfriend's graduation night less than a mile from her house. He was driving a convertible and hit a tree, causing her to be thrown out of the car. Her short life continues to be a reminder to me that life is a gift that we need to appreciate each day. I make it a point to visit her grave whenever I am in town.

I had a few special girl friends in high school and one special guy who was, and is, like a brother to me. Then, I could talk to him about almost anything. Well, almost anything. But because he never had a sister, there were some limitations. He was smart, creative, and talkative in a good way, and possessed both sensitivity and depth. We both went off to college, kept in touch throughout those years, and remain friends today. He was always such a philosophical guy. I remember sitting with him after we had put up all the decorations for graduation and having this long conversation about careers and destinations and what life had in store for each of us. Now, fifty years later, we are still having similar discussions, but now we are on the other side of life. It seems to come as quickly as the flip of a coin, and when you get to that point, you never know how many coin flips are left. It is truly a crapshoot. Ironically, his second wife died of multiple sclerosis.

By the time I graduated from high school, the very town that I was once so vexed about entering, I could not imagine ever leaving. In every way, this was home to me, and it felt as if I had never lived anywhere else.

At high school graduation, everyone's emotions are truly across the board from "Oh, yeah, I'm done!' to "Oh, shoot, wish I had studied more." I was surprisingly sentimental about the thought of leaving my high school and at the same time excited about the next chapter. One of my classmates had lost his mom the day before graduation. Just imagine what that was like for him. Another classmate had a dad who was very ill, while another, who had come to our town from Alabama to live with a host family, would return to his home state following graduation. It would be more than forty years before we saw him again. And, finally, one of our classmates, an unusual boy who often made funny noises in class and clearly marched to his own beat, would never be seen again. Less than a year after he graduated, he ended his life. Surely the problems of today were also the problems of yesterday, and today the world still struggles to find resolve in all this. It warmed my heart to know that his classmates, all of us, had embraced him all those years and tried to make him feel at home. What none of us ever considered was how scary the next chapter would be for him. Perhaps unable to find the support system that was afforded to him throughout high school, he decided to pass on it altogether.

As we all filed in to *Pomp and Circumstance*, my mind quickly flashed back to the day when my parents told me that we were moving to what was then a very small country town. I had felt completely unhinged. My whole world had unraveled. As each of our classmates spoke, I sat there feeling great pride being part of this amazing class. Not unlike the high school kids of today, as diverse as we were, we shared a special bond, a bond that would last well beyond our graduation day.

That day I remember looking out at my Latin teacher and recalling the first time he dressed up in his toga. I had to work hard to suppress a giggle. Even our seventh-grade home economics teacher attended. She once had the dubious honor of teaching me how to make an apron. As our eyes met, I am sure she was thinking, "My God, I cannot imagine anyone wearing the apron that child made." Late in the ceremony, I saw Madame Professeur reach into her purse, getting her cigarette ready to light up as soon as the festivities were over. When our eyes met, she put her finger over her mouth as if to say, "Don't you dare tell," since we were sworn to secrecy all the years that she had smoked in class. How I loved that woman!

What we had worked so hard for all those years was nearly over. The words to the song our class had chosen, "Somewhere," began. As we all sang "There's a place for us, a time and place for us …" I looked out at all the proud parents, so content that this milestone had been successfully achieved. Years later, in another state and in another high school, I would be one of those parents watching each of my own children graduate. And, if time allows, I will someday be attending my grandchildren's graduation.

High school was over. Time to party. Time for the next chapter. When you think about it, that is exactly what it's all about, a series of chapters in the book we call *life*. What I was unprepared for was how many years would pass before I once again walked those same halls, and that I would never again see many of my favorite teachers. It would be decades later when I finally returned.

Following graduation I was once again preparing to move on. I felt marooned, no longer connected to my high school and not yet in college. Many of my friends had dispersed for the summer and then would be off to college within days of returning; that would be the case for me as well. And if ever my parents could once again choose very poor timing to relocate, it was that summer. And where had they decided to move? Naturally, back to the place we had left all those years before. It certainly intensified the meaning of the word "transition" for me. To show how truly unsettled my dad was, they would eventually return to our small town one more time before they retired. It is for this reason that I have lived in the same town and the same house for several decades.

Moving On

College is a weirdly wonderful time of life. Mine was spent partly at an all-girls' college that had curfews and daily Catholic Mass requirements. It was in a setting that was much like the town I had first lived in: very urban and not far from New York City. What I was totally unprepared for was my freshman-year *roommate.* One minute she was lovely and the next very complicated and dark. I kept thinking to myself, "You have to be kidding me! I have to live with this?" It was going to be a *very* interesting year. It certainly did not make my entry into college life a warm and fuzzy one.

I was thankful that a high school classmate, who was also a good friend and hysterically funny, had decided to attend the same college. Her sense of humor was invaluable and I appreciated being able to use her room as my escape. Another landing spot was the smoker room. There was one on each floor of the dorm for those students who smoked. That is something you will not see in the dormitories of today, but in the 1960s they were everywhere. Within five minutes of arriving in the smoker room, your eyes would start to burn and even tear up. Sitting in a room filled with intelligent women, often playing bridge, each of whom had a cigarette hanging out of her mouth, was like a scene from both *Laverne and Shirley* and *Roseanne.* Although I didn't much like all the smoke, I enjoyed the distraction, as well as the socializing and the bridge tutorial.

On weekends, male students from the all-boys' college nearby would scale the building, threatening to come up to our rooms. But the nuns were better watch-dogs than any police canine team and quickly took care of that. On weekdays, we had an 11 o'clock curfew, when lights were to be out and the halls quiet. Never did we abide by that rule, so large groups of girls could be found hanging out in the private bathrooms that went with the singles to avoid the wrath of the nun who was in charge of the floor. Each time she came and knocked on the door, the same voice would have to respond with this brief reply, "Please, sister, I am having a problem and need to be in here for a while." It was all in good fun, and we enjoyed wonderful friendships with many of the nuns. They were dedicated professors who wanted to see all of us succeed.

My freshman-year roommate had talent that could have been epic: an operatic singing voice as well as fabulous acting skills, and she was successful academically, too. Sadly, when all was said and done, she did not make good personal choices in life. In the end, due to some very poor decisions, she was asked to leave the school. I then had the room all to myself and was happy to have a *somewhat* better roommate situation the next year, although at times her personal choices were equally perplexing.

Our college campus had once been owned by a New York banker who became a philanthropist and strong supporter of the Catholic Church. The land had a magnificent manor house replete with original artwork and period Roman statues from Italy that the owner collected during his travels. As a result, the arts were a very important part of our weekends and end-of-day activities, with many interesting offerings. I remember W. H. Auden coming for a poetry reading my freshman year. Visits by authors were common occurrences. I was also introduced to opera, today a true passion of mine. Although I was not a city person, I enjoyed being close to New York City and all that it had to offer.

Although some may take pause at the thought of an all-girls' college, I loved my classes, had fantastic professors, and made wonderful friends there. Today, all these years later, these classmates remain some of my dearest friends, with wonderful spouses and now fabulous adult children.

My dream to become a French teacher and live abroad someday was interrupted when, during the summer between my junior and senior years of college, I met the man who would become my husband. This guy seemed to come out of nowhere, and I was caught very much off-guard. Never did I dream that I would become a bride at the age of twenty-one. As provincial as it sounds, I never anticipated living anywhere but that wonderful town I had grown to love. I would soon live in a variety of places but never again in that bucolic spot.

Transitions

In many ways, this was a new chapter, both an exciting and a tumultuous time in my life. The war in Vietnam was going full throttle, and many of our friends were drafted and sent there. My own husband delayed graduate school and became an officer in the Navy, and fortunately was spared the perils of war. Those who went to Vietnam fought hard, and were lucky to return with all their limbs, but forever changed by what they saw. Some of our friends who were sent to Vietnam did not return. That was a wake-up call to many of us, perhaps foreshadowing the need for a bucket list.

Despite our becoming instant friends with many of the officers and enlisted men due to our shared circumstances, once my husband was discharged there seemed to be a total disconnect. Many of them were lifers, while we moved on to pursue our graduate degrees and to begin raising our families. I find it curious that in so many settings we meet people, connect with them almost instantly, and then, over the years, for really no reason other than the pace of life, gradually lose touch. Thankfully, today, social media have clearly bridged that gap.

Most unfortunately, I was doomed again to relocate, since we moved four times the first three years of our marriage. Childless in those early years, we never wanted for entertainment and were out almost every night, still rising early for our jobs. My preferred location was when my husband was stationed at the Pentagon and I was working in Chevy Chase, Maryland. An area that is dotted with museums and rich in history, it also provided the opportunity for memorable day trip options.

In spite of all my treasured memories of living there, on another level it was also the discouraging and racially charged 1970s, so we had front-row seats to the riots across the street from our garden apartment in Alexandria, Virginia. For a few weeks, I was actually escorted by a policeman to my car each morning, since he feared that I might find myself in the fray of the rioting when large rocks were thrown into people's car windows. It came as a result of the redistricting of two schools and the blending of two classes from each school. You would spend your freshman and sophomore years at one school and then be moved to the other school for your junior and senior years. It was a crazy way to integrate students and it came at a time when people were still reeling from the extreme prejudice that was so apparent not only in the South but all over our country. It made me sad then and it makes me even more sad today. And although this may sound like a stark contradiction to the reported racism that I witnessed at the time, in general, people did not seem to be as narcissistic as they are today, and the word transparency was never heard. We were coming off the "love" generation of the 1960s into what I always refer to as the "strange and still racially charged seventies," as people regrouped and tried to blend into a world that was moving on from a war, revisiting racism, and beckoning people to relocate and restart.

These were difficult times, and although there were also many exciting things happening in people's lives, the mood of discontent was very real and could not be ignored or perhaps I should say, should not have been ignored.

In spite of these events, I enjoyed living near the center of our government and we made many wonderful friends. But my best memory of those times was the day our son Breen was born and I became a mom. That gets top billing of any of the experiences we had while living there. Later I would have those experiences again, but in Boston, where our son Colin and daughter, Erin, were born.

I enjoyed all the places we moved to and the friends we made, but in the quiet of a moment, I still longed for my oldest and dearest friends. That being said, there was little time to reflect on that time in my life since it was all about family and getting your little ones through all the milestones. For some of us, it was also about completing graduate school and attempting to keep our sanity while doing all of the above.

We finally hung our hats up in a small town in Massachusetts, not far from Boston and close enough to the shore to enjoy a weekend getaway. One of my closest friends, who at the time was also my neighbor, would come to my house a few days a week at about four o'clock with her three kids in tow. It was the worst hour of the day to be with kids, but by putting her three and by then my three together to play in our fenced-in backyard for that last hour before dinner, we managed to find a good outlet for them and a little social hour for ourselves. We would sit there watching them play, sipping our one ounce of cream sherry on ice, engaging in our much-needed mom therapy. We also shared a similar sense of humor, and believe me, we needed it.

Today, there are all sorts of blogs and mom groups to do exactly what we accomplished in the hour we spent together in my backyard.

Back then we winged it, and when really in the dark, we would consult T. Berry Brazelton and Dr. Spock, who were known then as the experts with all the answers. Well, almost all.

A good chunk of my own time was spent getting our kids to their doctors' appointments, activities, playdates, and anything else that was required at the time. Our third child was born with congenital scoliosis, and so her journey was a bit bumpier than that of our two sons. We felt so fortunate to live in a medical mecca, where the required medical expertise could be provided on many levels, eventually leading to a successful outcome.

At the time, my husband had a demanding career that entailed a fair amount of travel and so I was often a one-man show. It was not unusual for a parent to come up to me and ask me how long I had been divorced. It always gave me a good laugh. I actually became the first PTO president at my children's elementary school who did not have a husband as her co-chair. That was actually a good thing, since it opened the door for single moms and dads to have the opportunity to chair.

Parenting during those middle, preadolescent years can be hair-raising to be sure. The ebb and flow of youthful hormones challenge the ebb and flow of our own hormones as we, reluctantly, approach middle age. You no sooner give a sigh of relief for having survived the middle years with your children than you find yourself experiencing their high school journeys. This is yet another chapter, dramatic as ever, often leaving you to wonder who really is in charge. It is not surprising that our salted and peppered hair so often emerges at this age and stage of life. In spite of all of the above, I enjoyed our children as emerging adults and I especially liked all their friends. As each of them began the college application process, it was truly daunting to think that they would soon be out on their own. It seemed as if in the blink of an eye they went from babies to biggies!

As you watch your children travel this journey through each level of their education, it feels as if they are mirroring your own school experiences, with mental images fleeting through your mind that surely bring you back to your own high school years. And then there are those times that you feel as if you are living vicariously through them, since the opportunities of today are clearly greater than those of yesterday. Today, they are living in an age of big data, able to communicate with friends on a level that was never an option for us. It is now nearly impossible to disconnect from your friends unless you are simply an anti-social person who prefers to keep to yourself. People now have the ability to find you, even if you might prefer not to be found.

The Wake-Up Call

AND SO, IN WHAT SEEMS like the blink of an eye, one by one the young ones leave the nest to pursue their own passions. No longer will you be racing to swim meets, soccer games, wrestling matches, basketball games, or tennis matches, or best of all, the many wonderful music and theatre productions that consume so much of their time. It suddenly occurs to you that for the first time in their lives, you will have no clue as to what they are doing and when they are doing it. You will soon learn what it is like to be starved for information. Any small nibble of communication from them is appreciated, and the realization that you now have a young adult in your midst is a dramatic nudge that you are aging.

Two years after my thirtieth high school reunion came the attack, the wake-up call that made me reassess what I wanted to do with the rest of my life. As I think back to that time in my life, never did I relate that dramatic nudge as the precursor to a medical journey of my own. All of my worries had been directed toward my children, never in my wildest dreams did it occur to me that my worries would soon flip to me. Eventually I would learn that other classmates were also confronted with medical journeys by the age of fifty, but at the time, I had been so wrapped up in my husband, my kids, my job, and my extended family and friends that it never occurred to me that life would throw me this curveball. It wasn't as if everyone I knew was healthy but rather that I felt fabulous and was a fairly athletically active adult who was more than aware of healthy living and eating habits. That's the trap that we all fall into. So often we don't see it coming because there are no red flags warning us that there is danger ahead.

After the attack, my high school soared to the top of my bucket list, although I was in quite a quandary as to how I would appropriate the time and energy needed to address it. I was teaching, as well as writing more and more, and had little time to think of a creative way to approach getting involved in anything, most especially a high school in another state. In spite of that, I would go on my computer late at night and surf high school alumni associations. Some of the websites were nothing short of extraordinary and often spearheaded by only a handful of alumni.

By the time my fortieth year out of high school arrived a decade later, I was on overload with teaching, writing, and working with a small committee to form an education foundation in our town. At the time, I was sitting on several boards, and almost every week I was off to meetings, each of which represented a cause that I was very passionate about. Finally, I decided to call a former classmate, someone I had become friends with that very first day at my new elementary school all those years ago. It was she who had a smile that could light up the world and she who rode the bus with me all through elementary, junior high, and high school. She was the mover and the shaker behind all our class reunions. Together, with a very small committee, we decided to do a Forty Plus One theme and have our fortieth reunion a year later. Little did we know at the time that more elaborate plans lay ahead for us. As our Forty Plus One reunion weekend was drawing to a close, I remember the wife of one of my classmates mentioning that it would soon be fifty years since our high school had first opened its doors. Hmmm. Fifty years. It became the daily buzzing in my head for many weeks to come.

My thoughts kept circling back to the idea of having all fifty classes gathering to commemorate and celebrate together. We needed to first find a way to open up the lines of communication so that we could eventually get regular updates on classmates and class events, and, of course, the much-dreaded news that a classmate had died. Lastly, there was the financial piece. Many alumni associations showed the students of today that the students of yesterday were paying it forward.

I suppose many, including some of my classmates, might wonder what the point of it all was. But just think about it for a moment. If you went to a good high school, as I did, it truly gave you legs to follow your dreams. If you went on to college or pursued additional training, it prepared you to stand on those legs. So many times the colleges are the recipients of all the good will, and the high schools are long forgotten. I wanted more for my high school, and I knew there was only one classmate who could help me pull this off.

I remember Googling my former high school to find out who the current principal was. I then called my old friend and classmate, who immediately came onboard, and suddenly we were off and running. The fact that there was no easy way of getting up-to-date information on alumni prior to 1980 surely complicated the task of finding people, and it would become one of our greatest challenges. Fortunately my co-chair, as well as a future committee member, knew exactly how to use the search engines to find people and how to create a website and Facebook page for them to find us.

We were in disbelief to learn that our much-loved and celebrated high school did not even *have* an alumni association. How could this be? It was a school that inspired so many accomplished adults. None of them chose to support a high school that continued to get some of the highest marks in the state. It was absolutely inconceivable to us, and, in time, my research suggested that this was true of many fine high schools.

Getting a high school alumni association off the ground is a mini-version of attempting to create a start-up company in the business world, equally labor-intensive but without any financial backing. The task needs to be addressed on a minute-to-minute, hour-to-hour, and day-to-day basis. Your mission is to reconnect and energize a population that is dealing with children, college loans, mortgages, busy careers, unemployment, aging parents, and perhaps medical issues of their own. You create your sales pitch, and you hope that they enjoyed the experience as much as you did and will want to buy in. Universities and colleges have development offices for this, while my high school would have two semi-retired women who didn't even reside in the town anymore and knew few people who still did. Fortunately, neither of us took each other too seriously, and yet we were very serious about getting both the event and the association off the ground. We were incredibly fortunate to find other alumni who quickly jumped onboard and shared our vision and our energy.

Now, imagine a busy high school principal getting a letter from a woman whom he has never laid eyes on offering to host a picnic for fifty classes on *his* watch, on *his* school property, needing help from *his* staff, and asking him to keep *his* school open to have the meetings in *his* conference room. Better yet, the event would be taking place two weeks before *his* high school students graduated.

Well, I would have to say that when it came to finding the right principal for all of the above, we hit pay dirt. He was and is nothing short of remarkable. As I sat there at our very first meeting, the thought occurred to me that he was not even born when I was in high school. My classmate and I were very impressed with him and with what he had accomplished. What was going on at our former high school was most inspiring and the accolades were hanging everywhere. The principal had a dry and quick wit, was a good businessman and a fine educator, and truly loved what he was doing.

When you go back to an old school after decades away, you see the amazing number of transformations that have taken place, from changes in the physical plant to the addition of high tech, as well as in the curriculum and the exciting course offerings that students of today have to choose from. Most impressive is the casualness that is part of the entire academic atmosphere now. This casualness is in and of itself a seeming contradiction to the competitiveness that is far more present in these times. You might call it relaxed competitiveness, a close relative of the oxymoron.

As you observe the modernization of learning spaces for students, you have to stand in awe of all that is now available to them. The resources foster future doctors, engineers, nurses, educators, businessmen and businesswomen, computer specialists and high-tech executives, as well as actors, musicians, photographers, jewelers, painters, and potters, not to mention the level of brain matter that fills each classroom, and the sophistication of the ideas that are shared. Lifelong learning is the new byline, and although that was true for many of us, it is now the gold standard for all. And if you happen to be athletically inclined, once again there is much to choose from, and the equipment is far better and safer than anything we ever had. Schools are very exciting places, and being back in mine reminded me of why I had decided to become an educator.

As we toured our high school and observed all the changes that had taken place, I was amazed to find my old locker. In my day, your locker was not only the place where you stored your books and winter gear; it was where you hung out, it was where you might find a box of chocolates on Valentine's Day or an unexpected note from an admirer. I stood there for a brief moment thinking back over all those years. It put a smile on my face as I opened the locker and realized it was a bit rustier but still had someone's schedule taped to the inside of the door, as well as some friendly graffiti. It also still pinched my finger when I opened it. Ouch! No one could ever fix that!

Our newly formed alumni committee was nothing short of amazing. We were a small group, but we all shared the same goal and were on a mission to see it happen. Some of our committee members who had graduated in the very first few classes had never had a reunion. It was unimaginable to my co-chair and me how many people who lived right there in the town had never considered an all-class alumni event. In truth, for me it was a dream realized, and I think that was also true for my co-chair. We enjoyed getting to know our committee members and appreciated both their energy and enthusiasm for what we hoped to accomplish. And as I reflect on those early meetings, I am not sure what was more entertaining: getting to know the principal, the staff, and our committee members, or reminiscing and listening to old stories that filled the room with moments of raucous laughter. It didn't seem to matter what year you graduated; every class had its favorite tales and they were surely worth repeating.

As we bantered among ourselves about high school reunions, we all agreed that they are very interesting events and take on a life of their own. No matter what high school you attended, or where it was located, reunion conversations are very predictable, and center on the decade you shared.

For example, as I think back to our thirtieth reunion, we were all in our late forties then, and many classmates had already achieved their goals in life. For some, financial solvency came and went during the recession of the late 1980s and ended in the early 1990s. Some classmates who had amazing leadership qualities in high school were unable to sustain them into their adult life, often through no fault of their own. And then there were those who, to the surprise of some, had found success and leadership skills far beyond what anyone would have envisioned. Then, when we gathered some ten-plus years later at our next reunion, the divorce rate had soared and many classmates were introducing the new replacement, spouse number two. In some cases, classmates had remained an item after high school, married, divorced, and ended up with another high school classmate, still keeping it as part of the same experience all those years later. To their credit, everyone seemed to remain on good terms. Then there were those who went off to college and at some point in their lives married, but it was not a good match; those who were successfully or maybe not so successfully still hitched; and those who were just beginning to contemplate sharing a life. Finally, for some, marriage was not in the cards.

The aging process operates almost like a barometer to the conversation as classmates reported their highs and their lows. Most perplexing and eye-opening was the prevalence of health issues, as many of our classmates were struggling with a variety of diagnoses. Some were on oxygen, while others had undergone extensive chemotherapy, with the hope of healthier days, and some, like me, quietly prayed for a slow progression.

As our very first meeting came to a close, my co-chair and I knew that we had not only a great committee but also wonderful support from the school itself. And as I drove back down the driveway, I felt as if I was home again, and as if time had stood still. It may have taken forty-two years to get there, but, finally, I was back.

Social Media

ON AN ALMOST DAILY BASIS my co-chair would find alumni and put them into our data base. It was all about finding as many people as we could, while leaving ourselves less than a year to do it all. Wisely, my co-chair made it a point to search the obituaries across the country. It was always with a heavy heart that we would add a new person to our list of deceased, a list that was growing far too quickly. It was at these times that we realized the timeliness of our mission. In our own class, we had lost about 5 percent to illness and accidents. That number would exceed 11 percent by our Forty Plus One Reunion, and continue to grow. I was grateful that I was still vertical and not being viewed in a box, a thought that was absolutely foreign to me all those years ago when I graduated.

The pendulum was now swinging in a new direction and, after years of yearning and an amazing amount of work, the important day had finally arrived, the day of the all-class reunion. The weather was totally uncooperative, but in spite of the raw chill in the air, we had warm hearts, smiling faces, and a very energized group of alumni who were like sponges for information. As I watched everyone being serenaded by the high school jazz band and a D.J., with frumpy clowns and face painters attending to the children, it soon became clear to me the alumni had become each other's entertainment, as one could hear raucous laughter coming from several areas of the field, not unlike how it used to be all those years before. Confessions were made in regard to failed relationships and friendships, and what seemed to be so important all those years ago was now a happy memory. Those alumni, who during their high school years seemed to be somewhat self-infatuated, were now mature adults with amazing experiences to share. Best of all, they were now interested in your story and not just in sharing theirs. As one alumnus reminded me, high school is truly a microcosm of life.

It is never really a reunion without once again reflecting on the various senior pranks that we had all been privy to. Surely everyone has a memory from their own high school days: from putting "for sale" signs on school roofs with phone numbers for interested parties to call, to rafting across a high school pond that had warnings to stay ashore, to encircling flagpoles with tires, to putting someone's outhouse in the senior courtyard, to any number of other creative surprises that make a principal's Monday morning feel more like an exhausting Friday. My all-time favorite was the time a cow was brought inside our senior courtyard, easy to do with a one-story, flat-roof building. By Monday morning, our principal had a fabulous panoramic view of the courtyard, full of cow plops, with a big cow staring him in the face while serenading him with morning moos. The cow was quickly escorted through the principal's office, down the hall, and out the front door to a waiting truck. The cow had evidently been borrowed from a nearby farm and may have been the first bovine to attend our high school.

I sometimes wonder what my life would have been like if I had stayed in the town of my early years, even though I truly love my life and cannot imagine living anywhere else. Surely, I would be penning another story!

Some of my classmates did just that, and now, years later, had children of their own who had attended our high school and were now alumni. Because we were a bedroom community to New York, the town had become a modern-day magnet for the rich and the famous, and for some, their time in my hometown was short-lived, often only to get their kids a good education, and then it was back to the Big Apple or wherever else they came from. For others, this bucolic setting fostered their creative spirit and they stayed for the duration. For sure, the real appreciation of where they were living came from the locals, who knew the history of the area going back to the Revolutionary War. The locals were and still are the real raconteurs.

Some of my classmates were the product of second-and third-generation immigrants who had arrived in these small towns, worked tirelessly, and became CEOs of successful companies and other local businesses, then passed on their work ethic to their children. Some were in the arts and were the offspring of composers and musicians, writers, and fine artists who followed the same path in their own careers. Many were small-business owners who had inherited their entrepreneurial skills from their parents. And many had created their own opportunities and entered any number of fields. For sure, it was an eclectic group of people, all of whom had a story to tell about what had brought them to these towns.

Reflections

The moment was bittersweet. What for years had been a mere phrase scribbled on my bucket list was almost over. A chilly drizzle was falling, as classmates were packing up and getting ready to return to reality. All the embraces and noisy greetings that had occurred just hours earlier were now emotional farewell hugs, as people frantically got that last selfie. I had spent a good amount of the day just looking down at all the faces I had not seen in far too many years. It warmed my heart to know that, together with our wonderful committee, we had actually pulled this off. Now we had a more seasoned yearbook face to relate to, and most importantly, a life update. So many alumni lived within miles of each other and yet had never crossed paths. At long last, our high school would have an active alumni association. Most important, we now had a number of ways to ensure that the connections could and would continue. Finally, it was all in place.

I am sure for some it was just like any other day, but for many of our committee members and most especially my co-chair and me, it was and always would be "The Reunion of All Reunions." Merriam-Webster defines the word reunion as "an act of getting people together again after they have been apart: an act of reuniting." I think we would define it as successfully searching, finding, connecting, energizing, and embracing those who knew us way back when, and reliving stories that had been dormant in our minds for far too long. It also allowed us to honor those who were no longer with us. Most of all, it was our way of celebrating an amazing high school and ensuring that there would be many more all-class reunions, at least for the remainder of our lifetimes, and hopefully beyond.

When I was a teenager, the concept of a "bucket list" was certainly not on my radar screen or anyone else's for that matter. Many aging parents had a wish list of things that they either hoped to do or wished they had done, but never was it described as a bucket list. While still a high school student, all those years ago, I had scratched three things on a piece of paper that I carried in my wallet and eventually stowed in my jewelry box. I'm not even sure what made me keep it. Perhaps it was a sign of what was to come. What I do remember very clearly is the morning of my attack when, as quickly as the click of a camera lens, my whole life flashed before me. At the time, it surely fit the parameters of multiple sclerosis. Without a doubt, it was the moment of reckoning that made me reassess my entire life, since I knew that it might never be the same again.

What I experienced emotionally at the time is experienced by any number of people who just like me, as a result of an accident, medical event, or diagnosis, realize that they are living in a different body, far different from the one they started with. The speed with which it sometimes happens is incomprehensible, but as I always say, like it or not, it is what it is.

I made the decision early on to be proactive, and I opted for the much-loathed lumbar puncture so that my doctor, a neurologist specializing in M.S. (very important), could get the spinal fluid needed to confirm the diagnosis. I actually insisted on it. Although you hear a number of negative stories regarding lumbar punctures, my experience was a very good one, and all I really felt were a few small needle pricks to anesthesize the area and a very slight bit of pressure. If you listen to your doctor and lie low for a week, it is a very tolerable process. I actually wrote my second book while recovering from my lumbar puncture, lying on a couch with my computer on my lap. It became and is one of my best-selling works.

There were no surprises when the results were in, no longer would my initials, M.S., stand for my maiden name, Mary Sunderland. They now took on a whole new identity: I had joined the much-dreaded M.S. Club.

Everyone reacts differently when given a medical diagnosis. After mine, I felt relief that it was me and not one of my children. I had the need to process it with two people who had always been there for me, my two cousins. One lived in a neighboring town and was experiencing her own health journey, while the other was in Kansas. I remember early on flying to Kansas and sitting on the floor of my cousin's living room, combing through every M.S. book that could be found on the shelf of a bookstore. I found the books less than uplifting, and actually, in many cases, somewhat negative. I knew where I had been but, at the time, I was not at all emotionally ready to hear about where I might be going. We finally put the books back in the bag and decided that they were in many respects, at least for me, not very helpful. I learned to rely on my medical team for updated information, as I continue to do today.

It was then that I decided that perhaps at some future time I would share my own journey. I must confess that never did I dream it would be presented in the context of a reunion. As I reflect on that decision, I realize that in many respects I needed all of these last seventeen years to assimilate and negotiate with myself as to how I would approach such a task and share the lessons I had learned. I wanted to be sure to convey to young adults just beginning their own journey that we cannot waste a minute, life is very precious, as well to suggest to those for whom this is new that we do not have to become our diagnosis. I think it is quite amazing that I am completing this manuscript just weeks after the fiftieth anniversary of the day I graduated from my high school.

One of the first lessons I learned right after I was diagnosed was that sharing medical conditions with those who fill your life can be a tricky journey, since most people have this stereotypical notion of how you might end up before they even know how you are doing. I am sure we have all been witness to what comes out of people's mouths when they greet someone who might be newly diagnosed, "How arrrrre you doing?" That is so not me, so I chose to take the high road, and with few exceptions, kept it to myself. That being said, I could always tell when someone knew, since they would sometimes give me this very subtle once-over, as if they were looking for something but were not sure quite what. I was not imagining this. On the contrary, others with the same diagnosis have shared that very same insight with me many times. Perhaps people don't even realize they are doing it. Surely they mean well. Maybe we should all wear signs, "doing well today," and for a bad day, "could be better." And when we get really progressive, "can't get much worse!"

Every once in a while someone who was privy to the diagnosis would express some momentary doubt regarding it and say, "Are you sure this is what you have? Maybe the doctor made a mistake." I loved all of them and was complimented by their momentary doubt. That's perhaps why they call it relapsing and remitting multiple sclerosis. There was no mistake: I definitely had it. I was more than aware of where I might be going, but I always loved that wonderful southern proverb, "Church ain't over until the fat lady sings."

Today, all these years later, newly diagnosed patients sometimes ask me how I felt emotionally when I learned the news of my own diagnosis. Quite honestly, I felt as if I had been catapulted into the air, and while in midflight, had this tiny window to reflect on everything I wanted to accomplish before I came back down to reality. Although it was certainly not something I had anticipated, it was most definitely a reality check for me. In hindsight, it is one that I am oddly thankful for.

My emotions ran the gamut: pain, fear, sadness, relief, and finally, determination. Whatever your medical diagnosis, everyone has his or her own way of dealing with it. Unquestionably, it is often a time of great uncertainty for all of us as we attempt to find our way. It is like going to MapQuest and not having an exact destination. You know where you are but have no idea of where you are going, emotionally or physically. Even more complicating is how you have to maneuver around your family as they deal with the diagnosis. At times, that can be quite exhausting, since we all want to protect our loved ones, some of whom do not always do well with medical information. And as I pen my own story, sadly, a significant number of people that I care about have just been diagnosed with some medical condition or disease, and are now experiencing their own roller coaster of emotions. I feel their pain, but most of all, I hope my story encourages them to look beyond their diagnosis and pursue their own bucket list.

For so many years I have remained silent, for the most part, in regard to my disease. As time passed, it occurred to me that some people might regard my silence as perhaps a discomfort on my part. On the contrary: I merely wanted the opportunity to live my life just like everyone else, one day at a time. Now, seventeen years later, I have decided that perhaps it is time to disclose the diagnosis so that I can share my own perspective on having M.S. In doing so, I see that my reconnection to my high school came as a result of my diagnosis, as did the actualization of a number of other line items on my bucket list. Although there are some things on my list that will be forever dormant, I believe that may be true for even the healthiest person. Hopefully, we can all look forward to and enjoy the things that we *can* continue to do, knowing that for some that list is unfairly very short.

Multiple Sclerosis

FOR THOSE OF YOU WHO do not know, multiple sclerosis is a neurodegenerative disease of the central nervous system. Today, 400,000 people in the United States have M.S. and 2.3 million worldwide, a daunting figure for sure. The initial attacks or physical experiences that might suggest that something is not right can be anything from a minor weakness, to numbness, to tripping and falling, and so on. The wrath of M.S. seems to have no boundaries.

Magnetic Resonance Imaging (MRI) is used to see how many lesions are in the brain or spinal area and that is often the barometer to the progressiveness of the disease. Beware! You can have an MRI that shows all is status quo and still have a relapse. Like many other autoimmune disorders, M.S. can be totally in control of your body. If you are like me and prefer to view the glass as half full, it means you are never alone, but without question, it is not quite the buddy you wished for.

When I was diagnosed, I experienced this wrath firsthand. The level of fatigue I felt was so overwhelming that I thought my body had simply given up on me. Since prior to my attack I was the energizer bunny, in time I managed to function relatively well in spite of the fatigue, but surely had to push hard to get through my workday. I have to admit that the initial experience of feeling as if every nerve on the right side of my body was on a rampage gave the term "tactile defensive" a whole new meaning, one that I will never forget. It was a totally inexplicable form of pain.

After an attack, the residual effects on your body can be anything from severe pain, to the loss of mobility, to incoherent speech and word retrieval difficulties, to numbness and tingling, extreme fatigue, and sometimes, to very few apparent changes. For me it involved about six months of napping to finally get through a normal day. Since I was working at the time, I easily slept right through my dinner for several weeks, and it was not unusual for me to be eating dinner at almost nine o'clock. A residual tingling and numbness lingered in my right leg for some time, often preventing me from getting a good night's sleep. I also experienced some temporary difficulty with word retrieval, but within a few months that righted itself. Since I was teaching, I worked hard to mask the symptoms, and did so fairly successfully. I had a tendency to lose my grip on things I was holding, some precious like an antique family dish, suddenly shattered on the floor. I referred to it as another "drama drop" as I stood there totally baffled as to how such a thing could happen so quickly and without warning. Thankfully, I have a better grip these days.

As one rebounds both emotionally and physically from the initial attack, that lingering worry persists that perhaps another might follow and manifest itself in another part of your body. Subtle reminders surface from time to time that affect your balance and coordination, often coming without warning. Only recently I lost my balance in my office, to find my head in a box of books and my legs where my head should have been. For the first time ever, I found myself laughing in a box! A good sense of humor is invaluable, but that is true even for the healthiest person. We are sometimes our own best audience.

Undoubtedly, the level of suffering for many people who have M.S. and many other medical conditions can be extreme and life-altering on many levels. We can only admire their courage and determination as they hope for remission or the "magic treatment" that will not only extend their lives but minimize the pain. Some have undergone extensive chemotherapy while others become wheelchair-bound and continue to function very well in spite of their condition. With the support of wonderful family and good friends and excellent medical intervention, they inspire those of us who know that someday we may well be where they are. And undoubtedly, our best role models when it comes to challenging health journeys, who surely put it all in perspective for people like me, are the many children who fight hard and never lose hope.

The buck doesn't always stop with M.S. Some of us have learned that although our M.S. journey is comparatively benign, other medical conditions may also knock on our door. In addition to all of the above, some of us have a whole new mantra created by the aging process: so many surprises, so few clues. We all need to stand strong and stay positive. Good nutrition, a daily workout program, setting goals, and a positive attitude all make these medical journeys more tolerable. Most of all, it is important to surround yourself with people who are trustworthy and supportive, and will not add to what is already a complicated diagnosis. Stress and M.S., as well as many other medical conditions, do not do well together.

Like many autoimmune diseases, M.S. is indeed a very individual journey, and sometimes the anticipation is worse than the actual trip. My best advice to someone who is newly diagnosed with any condition is to make friends with it by listening to your body. In time, you will get the hints, and in so doing, sort out what works for you. You may be able to live your life with few changes, all of which depends on how the disease or condition manifests itself. Even more important is how you, personally, deal with the diagnosis. As someone recently pointed out to me, I viewed my diagnosis as an opportunity and not a curse. It is just one chapter out of many, with more to come. It does not define who I am but has become my uninvited sidekick.

Whatever your medical condition or disease, treatment is personal to each patient. When it concerns M.S., I will say that much progress has been made in this area and there is a smorgasbord of options today that were not available twenty-five years ago. Multiple sclerosis researchers are hard at work and conferences are held regularly, with the best and the brightest leading the charge and showcasing what is available. I am told that remyelination is an area of active investigation, both in academia and in the pharmaceutical industry. There are several other areas being studied, including understanding neurodegeneration/progression and primary prevention in M.S. When you are considering treatment, I would strongly suggest that you rely on your neurologist. If in doubt, a good neurologist who specializes in M.S. will never be offended if you seek out a second opinion. Remember, this is your body and there are no dress rehearsals with M.S. or, for that matter, any other diagnosis. Please do not put off treatment, since it may be a missed opportunity. You want to do all that you can to keep the disease at bay.

I am more than aware that I have been, to date, very fortunate, and that I have not experienced the wrath of this disease more than that one time, with some very unpleasant hints that it could be returning for another visit. Many people who have M.S., as well as many other medical conditions, suffer on a daily basis, and their journey is far more complicated than mine. As is true of so many diseases, they have yet to find a cure for M.S. Researchers continue to explore any number of possible causes, such as low vitamin D levels, all of which are showing positive results in the lab. There is some discussion about the Epstein-Barr virus (EBV) making one more susceptible to M.S., but as yet there appears to be no definitive documentation of this. In my case, it was discovered that I am extremely low on vitamin D and this may have contributed to my own M.S. diagnosis, but this is only one of many possibilities. Many theories continue to be explored within the research community.

As I rewind the film of my own life, I did have a few clues before my attack that may have been a sign, but at the time I credited them to daily living. If I was under stress, the clues became more apparent, but still, I did not attribute them to anything of a larger scale. Only months before my attack, I began dropping things and also experienced some unusual urinary retention that I ascribed to not drinking enough water. Although the lack of water had nothing to do with it, today I am seldom without a bottle or glass of water in my hand. Perhaps the water has become my security blanket, but surely it has no impact on when my next attack may come.

For all of us who have been diagnosed with any number of medical conditions, there are some very important research opportunities available that often involve simply the donation of vials of blood. I encourage you to consider being part of that research, since it could significantly influence the possibility of a cure. It can be done in any number of ways and does not always have to involve a big wallet. If not for us, it may have a significant impact on those who come after us. It takes so little time and is truly paramount to finding cures.

So many medical conditions cause us to give up things that we enjoy, and for sure, none of us like to do this. These don't have to be losses, but perhaps an opportunity to review your options and find something new. I think of it as looking at life through new lenses. For me, viewing these changes as losses will only exacerbate what can become at any time a more complicated journey.

About a year ago I was diagnosed with thyroid cancer. Oddly enough, it was the good fortune of my annual MRI for my M.S. that provided an x-ray technician with the view of my thyroid that literally rescued me from a more advanced form of thyroid cancer. Thankfully, it was a very routine and successful surgery, with a good outcome. Had I not had that MRI, the cancer would have been far more advanced when found. This is another reason to look at the glass as half full.

I continue to walk four miles about three times a week and do a daily Pilates workout that a physical therapist designed for me. I also play eighteen holes of not very good golf twice a week in summer. Although I love to ski, it requires a lot of balance and quick turning. I did ski very successfully for several years after my attack, the last time in 2006. Now, well into my 60s, I prefer snowshoeing, because it allows me to still enjoy the beauty of a fresh snow with a more controlled gait. That being said, if there is a snowpocalypse, I may just surprise everyone and attempt to ski with my grandchildren.

Living for today and experiencing the joyful moments in life are my main focus and perhaps now they will also become yours. I have had the good fortune of attending and dancing at all three of my children's weddings. I spent a day watching my only daughter try on wedding gowns and make her final choice, a daughter who had traveled her own medical journey many years earlier. I have been able to experience the birth of my three granddaughters, Ella, Charlotte, and Zoe, and can still roll and play silly games with them. And, finally, I have been able to actualize a significant portion of my bucket list. I look forward to many more active years and hopefully more grandchildren. But I am more than aware that, at any time, I may well become inactive. This is something we all face, since none of us know when the ride ends.

The Bucket List

MY BUCKET LIST HAS SURELY been central to much of what I have done in the last seventeen years. The amazing thing about a bucket list is that you can reach for the extraordinary and not simply the ordinary. Some of the things on my list would definitely make you smile, while others are a work in progress and keep me busy. And then there are those items on my list that I will have to experience vicariously through someone else. Most important for me is having the opportunity to give back and to reach out to help others. It was my M.S. diagnosis that helped me to actualize things that had been scribbled on a piece of paper back in 1966. What began as some words with numbers next to them has been added to, massaged, and finally, checked off.

As I pen this story, that very first all-class reunion is in the past, and as I reflect on the last seventeen years, unquestionably the true catalyst for "The Reunion" was my 1998 diagnosis with relapsing and remitting multiple sclerosis. I have chosen a very circuitous route to finally write about it. Quite honestly, had I not been diagnosed, I am not sure that I would have ever completed this item on my bucket list. For me, "The Reunion" and my M.S. have become kindred spirits. My M.S. diagnosis forced me to address my bucket list with *une joie de vivre* that has energized me almost on a daily basis. It forced me to do things that I had longed to accomplish for most of my life and, in so doing, I forged many new friendships. Most important, it served as a reminder that a bucket list is something that should not wait and should be addressed early on so that "your ship doesn't sail" before it is too late.

I continue to be involved in a number of institutions, all of which are very important to me, but by far, my involvement with my former high school remains at the very top of the list. Each June, I try to attend the awards assembly there and take pride in seeing three high school seniors receive their Joel Barlow High School Alumni Association scholarship awards. I continue to be impressed not only by the number of awards and accomplishments earned by the current student body, but by the fact that no longer are only scholars and athletes being recognized. Today, students are acknowledged for any number of things that contribute to the spirit of the school, a dramatic change from the 1960s. And in June 2014, once again alumni gathered on my high school field for the second all-class reunion, and soon we will be holding the third. We now have a very active alumni association, and we have also been the catalyst to other efforts to involve the alumni. We continue to explore a variety of venues to raise money for our alumni association fund. The 2017 Joel Barlow All-Class Reunion is approaching. It is no longer a one-day event but a whole weekend of activities that I hope will continue for many years to come.

I believe that you can accomplish anything if you want it badly enough and are willing to work hard and take a few risks and have a good sense of humor to buoy you up when the going gets tough. My life is far from perfect, and like you, there are things that I might have done differently. I prefer to look forward and not back. I am grateful for the wonderful life I have and for my family, especially my three amazing children and their spouses; my dear grandchildren; the young adults who have been part of my life and whom I continue to think of as my children; my wonderful mother, who passed away in July of 2015; my amazing friends; and now you, my readers. Most of all, I am thankful that I have been given this priceless gift of time.

I am especially grateful that I grew up in that little jewel of a town that provided me with everything I needed, and some things that I didn't even know that I needed. I received an incredible education, have some fabulous memories, and enjoyed the beauty of nature daily with many wonderful friends.

As I think about my own life and what I want to accomplish in my remaining time, one of my favorite quotes from the French philosopher Teilhard de Jardin comes to mind. "The most satisfying thing in life is to have been able to give a large part of one's self to others." To me, that is the essence of life, and there are any number of ways one can accomplish this, no matter how much or how little you have. No matter what age or stage of life you are in, please, don't waste a minute.

There are those who view their life as a comedy and then those who prefer to see it as a tragedy. Perhaps life is in truth a satire that embodies all of the above. I have my own unique and sometimes humorous way of looking at my own life that in no way undermines the journey of others. To me, life is all about resiliency and reaching out, enjoying the gift of laughter, and remaining stalwart as one experiences the many uninvited guests that challenge that resiliency.

For those of you who share my M.S. diagnosis, clearly this book is a rather unusual approach to a reflection on having the condition.

I am aware that the story you pen will be very different from mine. If you were looking for a lot of factual information on M.S., you won't find it here. I feel that it is a very personal journey that we travel and each is unique to the person who travels it. If I described in more detail my own journey, it might cause you to unnecessarily anticipate something that might never come your way. I learned early on to take one day at a time. I encourage you to pen your own thoughts, stay connected, listen to your body, and go to your M.S. team for the most updated information and possible treatment options. Like you, it is my hope that the day will come when perhaps a cure will be found, or perhaps a solution to alleviate the suffering not only of M.S. patients but of everyone who is experiencing the painful challenges of a medical condition.

As I contemplated writing about "The Reunion" and my M.S., it never entered my mind to separate the two. For me, there was a cause-and-effect relationship that needed to be recounted as one story. Most definitely, I considered the confusion my readers might experience as I diverged from a high school reunion to life with M.S. But as I thought about it, life is all about the unexpected and how we stray from the norm. Perhaps my story will inspire young readers to be more empathetic to friends and family members who are traveling their own medical journeys. I surely hope that it has energized you to consider making your own bucket list, sooner rather than later. Most of all, I hope that you will appreciate what a good high school education can do for a student. Perhaps it will inspire one of you to become an educator or to create an alumni association for your own high school, or to join ours.

For those of you who were just looking for a good read, I hope you have found a reason to take pause and assess your own life. Reach for the extraordinary and you may be pleasantly surprised. Get it all down now, and enjoy the journey as you make each line item on your own bucket list a reality. It could be something you want for yourself or something you would like to do for others. I feel whole when I can do for others, and so a good part of my own bucket list has been about giving back and hopefully making a difference. All it takes is a piece of paper and a pencil, some gumption, and perhaps a wonderful old friend to become your partner in crime.

For my classmates and fellow alumni who are reading this book, without you it would not have happened. Now we have traveled yet one more journey together, and I am sure some of my comments will make you smile. Perhaps this will become fodder for your own recounting.

I didn't write my bucket list because I thought I was leaving this world but mainly because I wanted to prioritize and reassess. Perhaps my M.S. diagnosis was a wake-up call to remind me that I needed to get going and get it all in. It made me finally take piano lessons at the age of sixty, focus more time on my own writing, ski on the slopes of the Italian Alps, and do a number of other things that I doubt I ever would have considered even contemplating, let alone trying. And it made me reconnect with old friends whom I had missed for far too many years. Most of all, it helped me find my way back to a high school and a town that became the inspiration for much of what I wanted to accomplish in my lifetime. And, finally, the unexpected bonus is the many new friends I have made as I work my way through a bucket list that I have yet to complete. Remember the great thing about a bucket list is that you can reach for the stars.

I realize now that the little piece of paper that I started with way back in 1966 foreshadowed what was to come. And finally, after all these years, it makes perfect sense.

When I am not writing, my special place is now a pond surrounded by fields as far as the eye can see, where I enjoy the serenity of a small Vermont town and the fact that it is much like the Redding that I knew all those years ago. And if I could go down by the brook and hash all this out with the frogs one last time, maybe they would tell me this was the plan for me all along.

As I said in the beginning, life is like an adventure park. Each person gets only one ticket to enter. Sometimes we are up for the ride, while other times we might prefer to pass. Once it starts, there is no getting off. It can be a wonderful ride, or scary as hell. Most important, we try to get it all in before closing time.

Mary Mahony

SUCCESS

To laugh often and love much,
to win the respect of intelligent persons,
and the affection of children;
to earn the approbation of honest critics
and endure the betrayal of false friends;
to appreciate beauty,
to find the best in others;
to give one's self;
to leave the world a bit better,
whether by a healthy child, a garden patch
or a redeemed social condition;
to have played and laughed with enthusiasm
and sung with exultation;
to know even one life has breathed easier
because you have lived
this is, to have succeeded.

Bessie A. Stanley, c. 1905
Attributed to Ralph Waldo Emerson

John Wesley's Rule

Do all the good you can,
By all the means you can,
In all the ways you can,
In all the places you can,
To all the people you can,
As long as ever you can.

Thank you for taking this journey with me. Fifty percent of the proceeds from the sale of each book will go to the Joel Barlow High School Alumni Association with the hope that my legacy will live on for future generations. It is a cause very dear to my heart.

About the Author

MARY SUNDERLAND MAHONY GREW UP in Westport, Connecticut and moved to Redding, Connecticut, in 1958. She graduated from Joel Barlow High School in 1966. After graduation, Mary lived in New Haven, Connecticut; New York City; Alexandria, Virginia; and finally settled down in a suburb of Boston, where she has resided with her husband, Kevin, for more than forty years. She is the mother of three amazing and happy children, who have careers of their own and are now all married. Mary is the proud grandmother of Ella, Charlotte, and Zoe, with hopefully more to come.

Mary has master's and CAES degrees in special education and was an elementary resource teacher for many years. She began writing in 1997, something her high school English teacher had suggested she consider in 1965. Mary was a founding member of the Belmont Foundation for Education and has served on various boards for both organizations and hospitals that support children.

In 2008, Mary was invited back to Redding Elementary School as a visiting author. In 2010, Mary and her classmate, Sharon Morrissey, along with a resourceful and conscientious committee, planned the first Joel Barlow High School All-Class Reunion celebrating the fiftieth anniversary of the opening of the school. It was held in June of

2011, at which time they also formed the Joel Barlow High School Alumni Association, which supports high school initiatives and grants annual scholarships to deserving seniors to put toward their college education.

Mary is all about her bucket list, making a difference, and celebrating each day.

Joel Barlow High School

Joel Barlow High School is located in Redding, Connecticut, and is currently ranked as one of the top high schools in the state of Connecticut, as it has been for some time. The former principal, Dr. Thomas McMorran, was Principal of the Year in the state of Connecticut in 2012 and was nominated for the national accolade. In the spring of 2015, Dr. McMorran was chosen to become the superintendent of schools for the Redding/Easton School Districts. To Mary, he will always be the amazing principal who helped her realize a dream.

Gina Pin, who was also instrumental in helping the alumni association with that first reunion, has been promoted and is the current principal of Joel Barlow High School and the assistant superintendent of schools for the Reading/Easton School Districts. Both Dr. McMorran and Ms. Gina Pin continue to lend their support to the Joel Barlow High School Alumni Association as well the most recent initiative, spearheaded by the Athletic department, the formation of the Joel Barlow Athletic Hall of Fame. We are grateful for their ongoing support and look forward to working with them for many years to come.

REDDING PRESS
BELMONT, MASSACHUSETTS

WWW.REDDINGPRESS.COM

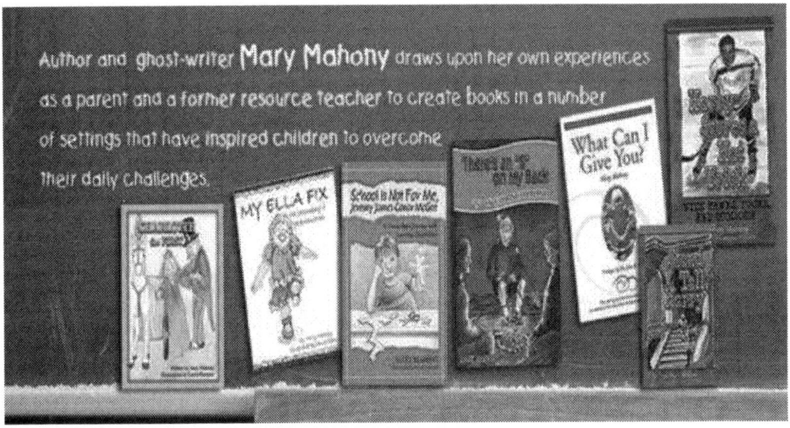
Author and ghost-writer Mary Mahony draws upon her own experiences as a parent and a former resource teacher to create books in a number of settings that have inspired children to overcome their daily challenges.
MY ELLA FIX
School is Not For Me,
What Can I Give You?

Made in United States
Orlando, FL
04 November 2026

90203420R00065